Ketogenic Diet

21 Days for Rapid Weight Loss, Increase your Energy And Live Healthy Lose Up To a Pound a Day

© **Copyright 2016 - All rights reserved.**

The contents of this book may not be reproduced, duplicated or transmitted without direct written permission from the author.

Under no circumstances will any legal responsibility or blame be held against the publisher for any reparation, damages, or monetary loss due to the information herein, either directly or indirectly.

Legal Notice:

This book is copyright protected. This is only for personal use. You cannot amend, distribute, sell, use, quote or paraphrase any part or the content within this book without the consent of the author.

Disclaimer Notice:

Please note the information contained within this document is for educational and entertainment purposes only. Every attempt has been made to provide accurate, up to date and reliable complete information. No warranties of any kind are expressed or implied. Readers acknowledge that the author is not engaging in the rendering of legal, financial, medical or professional advice. The content of this book has been derived from various sources. Please consult a licensed professional before attempting any techniques outlined in this book.

By reading this document, the reader agrees that under no circumstances are is the author responsible for any losses, direct or indirect, which are incurred as a result of the use of information contained within this document, including, but not limited to, — errors, omissions, or inaccuracies.

Table of Contents

INTRODUCTION	iii
CHAPTER 1: WHAT IS THE KETOGENIC DIET?	1
CHAPTER 2: BENEFITS OF THE KETOGENIC DIET	4
Fighting Cancer	4
Helps in Weight Loss	5
Treating Alzheimer's disease	6
Reducing Hunger and Cholesterol	7
Lower Blood Pressure	8
CHAPTER 3: COMMON MISTAKES TO AVOID	**9**
CHAPTER 4: FOODS TO EAT AND FOODS TO AVOID	**16**
CHAPTER 5: 21 DAY MEAL PLAN	**26**
CHAPTER 6: BREAKFAST RECIPES	**33**
Recipe #1: Pumpkin Pie Spiced Waffles	33
Recipe #2: Breakfast Cauliflower Waffles	35
Recipe #3: Cinnamon Sugar Donut Muffins	37
Recipe #4: Red Pepper, Bacon and Mozzarella Frittata	39
Recipe #5: Cinnamon Orange Scones	41
Recipe #6: Shakshuka (Eggs poached in a spiced tomato sauce)	43
Recipe # 7: Swiss Chard & Ricotta Muffins / Pie	45
Recipe # 8: Californian Chicken Omelet	47
Recipe # 9: Smoked Salmon Frittata	49
Recipe # 10: Turkey Breakfast Sausages	51
Recipe # 11: Breakfast Pizza Quiche	53
Recipe # 12: Cream Cheese Pumpkin Pancake	55
Recipe # 13: Bacon and Eggs	57
Recipe # 14: Lemon and Blueberry Muffins	59
Recipe # 15: Egg Muffin Cups	61
Recipe # 16: Choco Chia Pudding	63
Recipe # 17: Strawberry Chocolate Protein Shake	64
Recipe # 18: Cheese and Onion Quiche	65
CHAPTER 7: LUNCH/DINNER RECIPES	**67**
Recipe #1: Skillet Chicken Pot Pie	67
Recipe #2: Buffalo Chicken Jalapeno Popper Casserole	70
Recipe #3: Jalapeno Popper Soup	72
Recipe #4: Chicken Nuggets Served With Avocado Lime Dip	74
Recipe #5: Pepperoni Pizza	76
Recipe #6: Stuffed Poblano Peppers	78
Recipe #7: Crispy Curry Rubbed Chicken Thighs	80
Recipe #8: Cobb Salad	82
Recipe #9: Peri Peri Chicken Salad	84

Recipe # 10: Salmon Salad	85
Recipe # 11: Cream of Mushroom Soup	87
Recipe # 12: Chicken Soup	89
Recipe # 13: Beef and Vegetable Soup	91
Recipe # 14: Keto Beef Stir Fry	93
Recipe # 15: Ginger Beef	94
Recipe # 16: Baked Salmon	95
Recipe # 17: Spinach, Tomato, and Sardine Soup	96
Recipe # 18: Reuben Casserole	97
Recipe # 19: Butter Paneer Curry	99

CHAPTER 8: DESSERT RECIPES — 101

Recipe #1: Gelatin Pudding	101
Recipe #2: Coconut Oil Candies	103
Recipe #3: Berries and Whipped Coconut Cream	104
Recipe #4: Sugar-free Lemon Curd	105
Recipe #5: Brownie Cheese Cake	107
Recipe # 6: Chocolate Chip and Caramel Mini Muffins	109
Recipe # 7: Lemon Cheesecake	111

CHAPTER 9: LOW CARB SMOOTHIES — 112

Recipe # 1: Chocolate Peppermint Smoothie	112
Recipe # 2: Peanut Butter Smoothie	113
Recipe # 3: Sage and Strawberry Smoothie	114
Recipe # 4: Creamy Egg Smoothie	115
Recipe # 5: Raspberry Cheesecake Smoothie	116
Recipe # 6: Strawberries and Cream Smoothie	117
Recipe # 7: Choco-Orange Smoothie	118
Recipe # 8: Strawberry Chocolate Smoothie	119

CHAPTER 10: TIPS FOR LOSING WEIGHT — 120

Tip #1: Drink Enough Water	120
Tip #2: Fast Once In A While	120
Tip #3: Add Good Salts	121
Tip #4: Exercise	122
Tip #5: Avoid Too Much Protein	122
Tip #6: Choose What You Eat Wisely	123
Tip #7 Reduce Stress	123

CONCLUSION — 124

Introduction

A Ketogenic diet is a low-carb and high-fat diet. An individual following this diet regime reduces the carbohydrate content of his or her diet. However, the uniqueness of the program lies in its high fat content. Traditionally, avoiding fat-rich foods is considered the key to losing weight. This is perhaps the reason why we see so many foods advertised as 'fat-free' and 'low-fat' foods.

It is important to understand that when a food is devoid of its fat content, it has to include something else to maintain its palatable nature. In most cases, companies choose to add chemicals or sugar for this purpose. This makes matter even worse. Fats are not as bad as they are advertised to be. For instance, there are good fats that aid vitamin absorption, support organ functionality and facilitate healthy brain functioning.

Recent research has shown that an individual loses more weight on a low-carb diet than on low-fat diet. Besides this, the addition of good fats in the diet aids the body in many other ways, like lowing cardiovascular risk and improving cholesterol and blood pressure. Therefore, fats are not as disastrous as one would think and can be used to our advantage, particularly for improved health and weight loss.

A Ketogenic diet must typically contain as high as 75% fat. This is a huge chunk of the diet plan, and at first, you may actually find it hard to meet the fat requirements of this diet plan. Foods like cheese, butter, fish, nuts and red meats will become a permanent part of your diet. This is a complete shift in what we have been told to believe about these foods.

Before we move on to discussing Ketogenic foods and recipes, let us have a look at what 'ketogenic' means. The human body is accustomed to using carbohydrates as the fundamental source of energy and breaks them up using a process called glycolysis to generate energy. As a byproduct of this process, glucose is generated, which is then stored as fat in the body. Besides this, insulin levels of the body are also elevated during this process to facilitate fat storage.

This fat reserve is used only in situations when the body begins to starve. Considering the fact that our bodies rarely get into that state, these fat stores are really difficult to get rid of. On the other hand, when on a Ketogenic diet, the body is told to use fats as the fundamental source of energy. The process by which the body breaks up fats to generate energy is called ketosis. As a result of this process, ketone bodies are generated. The insulin levels of the body are also maintained during this process. This is specifically crucial for sufferers of diabetes.

There are several benefits of a Ketogenic diet. Some of these benefits include:

- Weight loss
- Stable cholesterol and blood pressure levels
- Maintaining insulin levels
- Reduced appetite

Apart from these health benefits, a Ketogenic diet also

improves the alertness levels of the body. A body that eats right will behave well. One of the best things about a Ketogenic diet is that you can be on a diet and still eat delicious recipes and mouthwatering desserts. So, starving is truly restricted to your body physiology. A Ketogenic diet, in no way, weakens you mentally or emotionally.

This book introduces some great recipes for your Ketogenic diet plan, which include recipes for breakfast, main course meals and desserts. Besides this, it also provides useful tips for making the diet plan work for you. We hope you use these tips and recipes to create a successful Ketogenic diet plan for yourself for in order to achieve a healthier and happier life.

Chapter 1:
What is the Ketogenic Diet?

Before I talk about the ketogenic diet, I want to give you an overview of a process called ketosis. This is a natural metabolic state that occurs when the body is lacking in glucose to use for energy, having to use stored fat instead – which is what we want to see. When these stored fats are broken down, they produce a stockpile of acids that are called ketones.

Two ways to get your body into this metabolic state are through starvation, which is not good for you, and a ketogenic diet. The idea behind a ketogenic diet is to stop your body relying on glucose for energy and force it into relying on your fat stores instead, hence the impressive weight losses recorded on ketogenic diets. The glucose comes from the carbohydrates that you eat and, by cutting them down severely, your body has no option but to look elsewhere for its energy.

The main sources of glucose are from starchy carbohydrates and sugars, like pasta, bread, rice, and potatoes. These are broken down, in the body into simple sugars and burned off as energy. What is not burned off will be stored as glycogen in the muscle and in the liver.

The Ketogenic Diet

The Ketogenic diet, sometimes termed ketosis or keto diet, is a low carbohydrate high fat diet. The ratios of calories consumed are about 75% from fat, 20% from protein and 5% from carbohydrates. Now, before you go off on one about the high fat level, let me just be clear on one thing – I am not talking about just any old fat. Later on, I will talk more about the types of fat you can eat and where to get it from but, for now, rest assured that there is, most definitely, such a thing as good fat. Basically, when you follow a ketogenic diet you severely cut carbohydrates and replace them with the right proteins and fats. Most of your carbohydrate consumption will come from vegetables and salad, with the rest of your macronutrients coming from meats, fish, eggs, and cheese.

There have been plenty of studies carried out on ketogenic diets and most have recorded similar result. One that was carried out on a group of obese men for a period of 4 weeks found that the average weight loss over that period was 12 lbs. All participants of the study found that they ate fewer calories but never felt hungry simply because they were eating the right kinds of food.

The Health Benefits of Ketogenic Diets

The ketogenic diet has also been shown to have significant positive effects on a number of serious and chronic health conditions, such as heart disease, metabolic syndrome, and diabetes, as well as improvements in levels of HDL cholesterol. This type of diet has also long been used by doctors to treat epilepsy in children with impressive results in the reduction of seizures.

Diabetes

The main condition that is affected by ketosis is diabetes. This condition occurs when a person does not have sufficient insulin to process all of the glucose they consume and if there are ketones in their urine it is a strong indicator that the condition is not being properly controlled.

Type 2 diabetes is the main one that benefits from a ketogenic diet. This is non-insulin dependent diabetes and this s because the body is still producing some insulin but can't utilize it properly. Because the ketogenic diet focuses on a reduction in carbohydrate intake, those with type 2 diabetes will benefit because it means that there is less glucose in their blood.

However, any diabetic who chooses to follow a ketogenic diet must seek medical advice first and they must undergo regular motoring of ketone levels. Although ketoacidosis is more prevalent in type 1 diabetes, those with type 2 are also at some risk.

I will be talking more about the benefits of the ketogenic diet in the next chapter.

Chapter 2:
Benefits of the Ketogenic Diet

The ketogenic diet is absolutely unique and it gives you benefits that you wouldn't find in any other diet. The main aim behind the diet is to reduce your dependence on carbohydrates and inducing your body to burn more fats.

Fighting Cancer

The ketogenic diet is a natural deterrent for cancer cells. The ketogenic diet usually consists of 75 percent fat, 20 percent protein and 5 percent carbohydrates. This limits the amount of carbs and sugar that you consume. Cancer cells replicate themselves throughout your body once they start growing. These cells need sugar in order to create enough energy to replicate themselves. Since, the ketogenic diet eliminates intake of sugar, the cancer cells are left stranded.

The diet also reduces your intake of carbohydrates. This further helps in fighting cancer, as the cancer cells do not have an alternative source to generate energy. This does not mean that you won't have the energy that you need for daily activities. Your regular cells can use fats to generate energy but cancer cells cannot simply switch to a different source.

Helps in Weight Loss

If we consume carbohydrates, insulin is released throughout the body in order to increase blood glucose. Insulin is a type of hormone. Its basic function is to ensure that the body has enough energy for all of its needs. So, when insulin is released it further propagates the cells to save as much energy as possible. The cells initially save the energy in the form of glycogen (carbohydrates in their stored form) then later on as fat.

The ketogenic diet aims at reducing the level of carbohydrates that you consume so that they are almost negligible in your body. This prevents your body from releasing insulin. When insulin is not released in the body then there is a lack of glycogen, which the body needs in order to generate energy. Hence, your body is forced to burn fats in order to generate energy. This helps in reducing the amount of fats that are stored in your body and therefore, helps you to lose weight.

Treating Alzheimer's disease

Alzheimer is a disease that slowly deteriorates your nervous system. If it goes untreated it can even lead to Dementia. The ketogenic diet is the perfect way to treat Alzheimer's.

When you get old, the nervous system stops working properly and tends to slow down after a while. This causes mood swings, random episodes of dementia and most importantly memory loss. To prevent Alzheimer's from growing, it's important to take care of your nervous system. The nervous system is directly linked to the brain. So, to help the brain it is important to consume healthy fats. Healthy fats make your brain more active. The ketogenic diet consists of 70 percent healthy fats and hence, it helps the brain.

It's also important for your brain to be able to burn fatty acids in order to gain energy. This helps in the treatment of dementia, as your brain is more active than before. So, the ketogenic diet helps you in the maintenance of your nervous system.

Reducing Hunger and Cholesterol

The ketogenic diet can be considered as a miracle because it actually reduces your hunger. If you are someone who tends to snack randomly and is not able to control his food consumption then the ketogenic diet ensures that you don't get too hungry too often.

The reason behind this is the consumption of fat. Fat is very satisfying and it makes you feel full for a longer period of time. If you suffer from food addiction issues then the ketogenic diet will make you feel great. There will be times that you might even skip meals without even realizing it.

The ketogenic diet also helps in reducing cholesterol in your body. Cholesterol is a fat like substance that is produced by your body and is also present in some foods that you consume. If produced in excess, cholesterol can be very harmful. Cholesterol is made when there is excessive glucose in your diet. If you consume foods with less sugar then your body will not have the glucose it requires to create Cholesterol. Hence, the cholesterol levels in your body will drop.

Lower Blood Pressure

Elevated blood pressure can lead to many diseases including heart attack, kidney failure and others. The ketogenic diet makes sure that you do not consumer too many carbs. This reduces the blood pressure of your body. It's been seen in numerous cases that a reduction in consumption of carbs led to decreased blood pressure. The reason behind this is that a low carb diet induces the body to store less fluid. This includes the constituent fluids present in blood. A lower blood pressure reduces the risk of an early death and also makes you feel more energetic than before.

In the next chapter, we will look at some of the more common mistakes that people make on ketogenic diets.

Chapter 3:
Common Mistakes to Avoid

The ketogenic diet is more of a lifestyle and, like any change you make in your life; it requires some getting used to. There is a lot to learn and you won't get it right first time, simply because everyone is different and we all have different needs. Some of these learning curves can lead to a great deal of disappointment and frustration as people don't see the results they expect to see as quickly as they want to. The following are the most common mistakes that people on a ketogenic diet make and how to fix them:

1. **An Obsession with Macros**

Macros are macronutrients and these are quite simply fat, protein and carbohydrate. The biggest mistake that people make is getting obsessive over their macros. One of the biggest benefits, psychologically speaking to the ketogenic diet, is the freedom that it offers. No more are your days tied to food. Instead, although you should track your macros let go of the obsession. It doesn't matter if you eat one percent less fat and two percent more protein. The idea is this – you are not eating macros, you are eating food, real food. Provided what you eat is keto-friendly, you will be doing absolutely fine.

2. **You Are Obsessed with Your Scales**

The single least important thing that you use to judge your progress and success is the number on your scales. So many people obsess over their progress that they get on the scales every single day, sometimes twice and then panic when their weight has gone up. First, your weight fluctuates on an hourly basis and every time you weigh yourself it is going to be a different number. Second you should only weigh yourself once per week. Do it at the same time every week, first thing in the morning and you will get a better reading of your weight loss. Third, life is for living not for standing on scales. Again, provided you are eating the right foods and are not cheating, your progress will become self-evident.

3. You Eat Too Much Protein

Protein is a very important macro simply because we cannot do with it. Protein is required for certain amino acids that the body cannot produce and it also provides the building blocks for soft tissues, like organs and muscle. However, if you eat too much of it, your body will not go into a state of ketosis. For every 100 g of protein that you eat, 56 g is turned into glucose so eating far more than you need to means more glucose is produced and that means your body will never need to burn off the fat for energy. One of the best things about the ketogenic diet is that it is "protein sparing" – this means that nutritional ketosis will hold the protein in your body and not strip it out like high carb foods so.

4. **You Are Not Eating Enough Fat**

So many people are afraid of fat that, even on a high fat diet they still don't eat enough. The problem here is that, over the years, we have been conditioned, even brain-washed to a certain extent, that fat is bad and, to get over that hurdle, it takes a great deal. All I can say here is trust in the fat because it is the fat that is going to put your body into ketosis and turn it into a fat-burning machine. And, if it is of any help, the human body has certain biochemical responses to dietary fat and provided you are eating good fats, you really can't eat too much so tuck in and enjoy. That leads to the next mistake.

5. **You Are Not Eating the Right Kind of Fat**

It's one thing eating loads of fat but you have to eat the right kind of fat. The worst ones are vegetable oils and seed oils, margarines and the fats found in baked and processed goods. These are not healthy and will sabotage all of your best effort. The right kind of fat is saturated and monounsaturated fat – coconut oil, olive oil, butter, animal fat, avocado, etc.

6. **You Eat Processed "Ketogenic" Food**

The idea of the ketogenic diet is to eat real whole food, not processed. If it comes in an individual wrapper, it isn't real food. There are plenty of these so-called keto snacks and all they will do is put a halt to your weight loss. They are not proper keto foods they are just a distraction. If you have to eat one on occasion, then that's OK but the majority of your diet should be real food that is made with real ingredients.

7. You Worry Too Much About Your Cholesterol

So many people believe that a high fat diet cause your cholesterol to go up. And, for many years you have been told that cholesterol is bad for you, that it is dangerous. Well, get this into your head – it a myth. Cholesterol is actually required by your body, by every single cell in your body. High cholesterol does not mean that you are at risk of heart attack or cardiovascular disease so there really is NOTHING TO WORRY ABOUT. One of the biggest reasons behind the worry is the diet-heart hypothesis put forward by Ancel Keys. He asserts that a high level of cholesterol, caused by too much saturated fat, will have a negative effect on your cardiovascular and heart health. There was no evidence to back up this assertion and later on down the line Keys actually rejected the hypothesis. Unfortunately, his original assertion is what made us scared of cholesterol in the first place. He rejected it and so can you.

8. You Want a Quick Fix Weight Loss Program

I really am not going to waste too much time on this one. The ketogenic diet is far from being a quick fix. It is a way of life. If you have it in your head that you can drop a few pounds quickly on the ketogenic diet and then resume your normal lifestyle without gaining it all back, think again this is not the diet for you if that is what you are looking for.

9. You Are Not Fully Committed

The ketogenic diet is not something you can go at in a half-hearted manner. You must be fully committed to it for the simple reason that it requires real determination. You are changing everything about the way you eat and you are choosing a lifestyle that the vast majority of society simply can't get their heads around. There is no sitting on the fence here – you cannot eat a high fat diet and high carbs as well. Not only will you pile the pounds on, it is actually a dangerous combination and a real risk to your health. Dive in fully committed and the results will speak for itself.

10. You Eat Because the Clock Says You Should

Really, no matter what you have been told over the years you don't have to have breakfast in the morning. You don't need to have your lunch just because it is noon and you don't need to eat dinner because the clock says it is 6 pm. You don't have to stop eating at a certain time and avoid eating at bedtime. This is something else that has been drummed into you over the years – to eat by the clock, not by your body. It's quite simple – eat when you are hungry, don't eat when you are not. If you are hungry at 10 pm, eat something. The clock on the wall has no relation to and knows nothing about the clock in your body and that is the clock you should be listening to. Your body will tell you when it is the right time to eat so learn to listen to it.

11. You Compare Yourself to Other People

Stop. Really, stop because everyone is different. How someone else progresses are not by any means an indication of you will progress on a ketogenic diet. You gain and lose fat in different places and in different ways to the person next to you. It's important to keep that in mind if you are trying to measure your success based on theirs. Just because Fred lost 100 lbs. in one month doesn't mean that you will and it doesn't mean that you have failed if you don't. Just because Simon dropped his body fat down to 10% doesn't mean that you will or that you have failed if you don't. Again we are all different and we all do things differently. Learn what works best for you and keep on doing it. The only thing that will NOT work is to keep on comparing yourself to other people.

12. You Are Not Getting Enough Vitamins and Minerals

In particular, I am talking about salt, magnesium, potassium and vitamin D. A salt imbalance is one of the biggest issues that anyone on a ketogenic diet will come across. We tend to avoid salt because it has a bad effect on a body that is already inflamed through an improper lifestyle. The trouble is, when you are on the ketogenic diet, your body is no longer inflamed and, as such, you need more salt. You should be adding at least 2 tsp. a day to your diet. You will also find that you are running short on vitamin D, potassium and magnesium so, if you don't get enough in the food you are eating, make sure you take a good quality supplement

13. You Are Trying to Do It Alone

When you make a huge change in your life, no matter what it is, you should never try and do it on your own. Have supportive people around you, people who can encourage you and get you through the worst days. Join a group on the Internet, a physical group or just have some good friends and family around you who understand your struggles, your success and the journey you are undertaking. You need someone to encourage, to admonish and to walk alongside you otherwise you will find it hard.

Chapter 4:
Foods to Eat and Foods to Avoid

So what can and can't you eat on a ketogenic diet. In simple terms, you should be eating real whole foods, such as meat, vegetables, fish, nuts, yogurt, and on occasion, fruit. Apart from the fact that you should be eating foods with little carb content, you should also avoid all processed foods and anything that contains colorings or preservatives.

The ketogenic diet is not just about the weight loss; it is about starting and maintaining a healthy lifestyle. Below I am going to list the best low-carb foods for the ketogenic diet along with pointers for what you can eat in moderation and what to avoid

Fats and Oils

These are going to be the vast majority of your caloric intake, so make your choices based on your own digestion system:

- Wild caught trout, salmon, tuna, mackerel, shellfish, etc.
- Butter, coconut butter, lard, ghee, beef tallow, chicken fat, duck fat, goose fat
- Macadamia nut oil, olive oil, coconut oil
- Avocados and avocado oil
- Mayonnaise
- Organic peanut butter

Avoid

- Margarine
- Vegetable oils
- Sunflower oil
- Anything with trans fats in it – processed foods

Nuts and Seeds

These should be consumed in moderation

- Almond
- Macadamia nuts
- Walnut
- Pine nuts
- Pumpkin seed
- Sunflower seed
- Cashew
- Pistachio
- Chia seed
- Flax seed
- Coconut

Substitute normal flour with almond flour, flaxseed flour etc.

Proteins

Try to stick to grass-fed, organic and free-range proteins:

- Fish – catfish, cod, halibut, flounder, snapper, trout, salmon, tuna, etc.
- Shellfish – oyster, clams, lobster, scallops, crab, squid, mussels
- Eggs
- Meat – beef, goat, lamb, veal
- Pork – loin, chops, ham – check for added sugar in ham
- Poultry – chicken, turkey, duck, goose, quail, pheasant
- Bacon/sausages – check for additives, sugar, fillers, etc.

Avoid

Anything that is processed, breaded, battered, etc.

Vegetables

The best vegetables are those that are grown above the ground and not below it and also dark leafy greens.

- Asparagus
- Broccoli
- Carrot
- Cauliflower
- Celery
- Garlic
- Cucumber
- Green beans
- Onion
- Mushrooms
- Bell peppers
- Dill pickles
- Lettuce
- Snow peas
- Spinach
- Kale
- Squash
- Tomato

Dairy

Go for free-range/pastured sources and choose full-fat versions instead of low-fat or no-fat:

- Cream
- Cheese – cheddar, gouda, edam, mascarpone, mozzarella, cream cheese, cottage cheese
- Full fat milk

Drinks

The ketogenic diet will have a natural diuretic effect on you so one of the things that you are likely to suffer from is dehydration. This is even more important if you are one of those that are prone to bladder or urinary tract infections.

The following are beverages that you can drink as much of as you want:

- Water – at least 2 liters per day. If you don't like plain water, add fresh lemon slices or cucumber to it
- Coffee – black or with cream
- Tea – black, green, herbal, fruit

Sweeteners

Your best option is to steer clear of anything that is sweet because it will help to control cravings – killing cravings is the best way to succeed on the ketogenic diet. If you do need something sweet, go for one of these sweeteners and choose the liquid version over powdered or granulated:

- Stevia
- Sucralose
- Xylitol
- Erythritol
- Mon fruit
- Agave – be cautious with this as it can be high in carbohydrate

Avoid anything that contains aspartame

Spices and Herbs

Spices are quite tricky because most spices contain carbs. It is important, therefore, that you add them into your daily carb count. Herbs can be eaten freely

- Sea salt
- Basil
- Black pepper
- Chili powder
- Cayenne
- Cilantro
- Cumin
- Parsley
- Oregano
- Rosemary
- Sage
- Turmeric
- Thyme

Avoid

Prepackaged spice that contains sugars, table salt and spicy sauces

What to Look Out For

Some foods are quite difficult when it comes to the ketogenic diet so be careful of these foods:

Spices

Some contain higher carb counts than others so avoid these if possible or heavily restrict your intake:

- Cinnamon
- Onion powder
- Garlic powder
- Bay leaf
- Allspice
- Cardamom
- Ginger

Fruits

To be fair, most fruit is prohibited on the ketogenic diet because of the sugar content. You can still eat the following but in small amounts only:

- Raspberry
- Strawberry
- Blueberry
- Cranberry

Tomato-Based

The reason I have listed these separately is because so many of us use them in the form of tinned tomatoes and sauces. However, these tend to be very high in sugar so always check the label and restrict your intake of them as much as possible. You can make your own tomato sauces out of natural ingredients, without the need to add in sugar.

Peppers

Believe it or not, these are also quite high in sugar so monitor your intake. Stick to green pepper as the red, orange and yellow ones are higher in carbohydrates.

Diet Drinks

You can drink these on the ketogenic diet but not to excess. Some people have said that after drinking a lot of diet drinks they have come out of ketosis and have had to start over again. There is a definite link between the artificial sweeteners in these drinks and sugar cravings as well so these drinks are likely to make life tougher for you.

Medicine

Medicines for colds, coughs, and flu medicines all contain carbohydrate in high levels. Some of the ones you can buy over the counter contain a whopping 20 g of carbohydrate in each serving so make sure you buy the sugar-free ones instead.

How to Control Your Cravings

When you first make the change to a ketogenic diet, cravings area going to be almost constant and they will almost certainly hit you out of nowhere at times. But this doesn't mean that you have to fall off the wagon for the sake of just one sugary treat.

When you get a craving, what your body is actually telling you is that it is low on a nutrient. Foods loaded with sugar and carbohydrate are not the only way to fulfill those cravings. The following list contains common cravings, the nutrient you are missing and what to eat instead:

Craving	Nutrient	What to Eat
Chocolate	Magnesium	Seeds, nuts
	Chromium	Cheese, broccoli
	Carbon	Spinach
Sugary Food	Phosphorous	Eggs, chicken, beef
	Sulfur	Broccoli,

Cauliflower

| | Tryptophan | Liver, lamb, cheese |

Carbs – bread,
 Pasta, etc.   Nitrogen   Meats high in protein
Oily or fatty foods   Calcium   Spinach, broccoli, cheese
Salty food   Chloride   Fish
                      Silicon   Seeds, nuts

So, now you know how to control your cravings, let's move on to how to set yourself up for a 21-day ketogenic diet plan.

Chapter 5:
21 Day Meal Plan

What does a good ketogenic diet plan actually look like? Well, there isn't any such thing as a plan, as it were. It is simply a case of picking a meal from each of the sections for breakfast, lunch, dinner, etc. and only eating that plus the proper snacks throughout the day. However, I have decided to give you an idea of a 21-day plan – you will find some meals are duplicated, but that is only for simplicity.

Before we look at your meals, let's take a look at how to set yourself up for success on the ketogenic diet:

Guidelines

We know that the ultimate goal of a ketogenic diet plan is to improve your health and with to burning fat through a metabolic process called ketosis. Before you begin a ketogenic diet, you should seek medical advice from your doctor particularly if you have diabetes, type 1 or 2, or any other medical condition. If you suffer from any disease of the kidneys you will need to be especially careful.

Basics of the Ketogenic Diet Plan

There are lots of ways to do a ketogenic diet, but all of them involve eating more fat and less carbohydrate. Many people confuse ketogenic diet with high protein diets but they are not the same thing. As we discussed earlier, too much protein can have a detrimental effect on your health. The following are the two basic rules of any ketogenic diet plan:

- Keep your carb amount to between 20 and 60 g per day and track what you are eating.
- Although counting calories is not so important, you should aim for about 70-75% of your caloric intake from fat 5-10% from carbohydrates and 20-25% from protein.

How to Start Your Ketogenic Diet Plan

- Get yourself a guide for counting carbs. You can get an app for your smartphone or tablet or you can use the Internet but this is a vital part of the diet plan.
- Sweep the house of carbohydrates. Look through your cupboards, refrigerator, and freezer and ditch any high carb food, including any of those so-called healthy whole grain foods. The less temptation there is, the more likely you are to be successful

- Restock. Now you can fill up your cupboards and freezer/fridge with low carb ingredients. That way, when you do get an urge to snack, it will be something that you are allowed to eat. You do not need to buy special low-carb packaged foods because this is not a special diet. Ketogenic foods are nothing more than real foods that are low in carbohydrates; in other word, foods that are not processed, with the exception of sweeteners should you choose to use them.

- Be prepared to do more cooking. Because you are going to be using real foods, you are going to be spending more time cooking instead of just tipping something out of a packet into a pan.

- Think about what you are going to be eating in advance and plan them properly. You need to make sure you buy the right foods and it also makes it easier when you know what you are meant to be eating

- Change your habits. If you usually stop off for coffee and a bagel on your way to work, make your own coffee at home and have some eggs with it.

- Make sure you stay fully hydrated. A low-carb diet pushes your kidneys into getting rid of excess water that used to be retained through eating a high-carb diet. This means that it is more important than ever that you replace the water you are losing. If you get cramps or headaches, you aren't drinking enough and you are also lacking in minerals like magnesium, salt, and potassium – when you eliminate water, those minerals go with it.

- Do make sure you avoid any high carb food that has the ability to drive your glucose and insulin levels way up. As well as that, cereal grains are highly toxic to some people, specifically wheat, and you may be dealing with an undiagnosed or untreated gluten intolerance

- One way to find out if you are in ketosis is to purchase ketostix from your pharmacy. For the first few weeks, the sticks are used to measure ketones in your urine and they should register a deep purple when you go into ketosis. After that, you should be keto-adapted and using up the ketones as energy so they do not register on the stix.

- Track your food and carbs daily. Write it all down or use a specially designed tracker on the Internet. This will help you to keep track of what you are eating, how you feel and what changes you make if something isn't working for you.

- Consider social situations. Come up with a plan to cope with meals out or at another person's house because if you don't, the temptation to eat high carb foods will be high.

- Don't focus only on your weight, even if that is what you started a ketogenic diet for. Forget weighing yourself daily because changes in your body and water absorption can mean a 2 to 4 lbs. difference every day. Instead, focus on how you feel. Weigh and measure yourself once a week and write everything down in your food journal or online tracker, including any off days you may have. You could also get a blood panel done so that you can track changes in your blood pressure, cholesterol, and other markers. After 4 to 8 weeks you can the same tests one and see what the differences are

- Learn how to deal with craving and stop sugar cravings in their tracks. There are other foods you can eat that will have exactly the same chemical effect on your body – you just need to know what they are

21-Day Meal Plan

Choose one meal from each of the lists for each day of the diet. You can also substitute dessert or lunch with a smoothie if you prefer. Repeat for 21 days, mixing up your meals so you don't get bored of eating the same thing. These are just idea for your meals so feel free to look around and choose other low-carb meals instead

Breakfast:

Pumpkin Pie Spiced Waffles

Cinnamon Sugar Donut Muffins

Breakfast Cauliflower Waffles

Choco-Chia Pudding

Cheese and onion Quiche

Bacon and Eggs

Red pepper, bacon and mozzarella frittata

Lunch

Jalapeno popper soup

Cobb salad

Cream of mushroom soup

Salmon salad

Chicken soup

Peri peri chicken salad

Spinach, tomato and sardine soup

Dinner

Skillet chicken potpie

Pepperoni pizza

Keto beef stir-fry

Buffalo chicken jalapeno popper casserole

Baked salmon

Butter paneer curry

Ginger beef

Dessert

Berries and whipped coconut cream

Lemon cheesecake

Sage and strawberry smoothie

Brownie cheesecake

Raspberry cheesecake smoothie

Gelatin pudding

Choco-orange smoothie.

Chapter 6:
Breakfast Recipes

The day starts with a breakfast and a delicious breakfast can set the right tone for the rest of the day. This chapter has five breakfast recipes that can be added to your ketogenic diet plan. You can try these simple recipes and vary them according to your personal taste. These can benefit you, both in terms of dietary benefits, and how delectable the recipes are.

Recipe #1: Pumpkin Pie Spiced Waffles

Serves – 2

Ingredients –

- 1/4 cup Canned Pumpkin
- 1/3 cup Coconut Milk
- 1 1/2 teaspoon Pumpkin Pie Spice
- 2 large Eggs
- 1 teaspoon Baking Powder
- 1 teaspoon Vanilla Extract
- 2 tablespoons Flaxseed Meal
- 7 drops Liquid Stevia
- 3 tablespoons Swerve Sweetener
- 1/2 cup Almond Flour

Instructions –

- Take a jug and mix in all the liquid Ingredients. Blend until any white component of the egg becomes visible.
- Take another container and mix all the dry Ingredients. Use a sifter to make a uniform mix.
- Mix in the dry Ingredients mix to the wet Ingredients mix. The consistency of the batter should be a little watery.
- Take the waffle maker and grease it with coconut oil. As and when the waffle iron becomes hot and ready for use, put the batter into the waffle iron.
- Remove the waffles as and when they are done.
- You can serve these waffles after spraying some maple spray and some pecans.

Recipe #2: Breakfast Cauliflower Waffles

Serves – 4

Ingredients -

- 3 Large Eggs
- 1/4 cup Parmesan Cheese
- 1/2 cup Mozzarella Cheese
- 1 cup Raw Cauliflower (grated)
- 1/2 cup Cheddar Cheese
- 1/4 teaspoon Red Pepper Flakes
- 1/2 teaspoon Garlic Powder
- 3 tablespoons Chives, chopped
- 1/2 teaspoon Onion Powder
- Pepper
- Salt
- Eggs Benedict – One Serving
    - 2 slices Prosciutto
    - 2 large Eggs
    - 2 tablespoons Hollandaise Sauce

Instructions -

- Before starting, get the cauliflower and chives ready for preparation.
- Using the grater, process the cheese and cauliflower together.
- Add the seasoning, chives and eggs to this grated mix.
- Prepare the waffle maker and when it is ready, put the grated mix to the waffle maker.
- Cook both the sides. This should not take more than 10 minutes.
- In order to make the topping of single serving eggs benedict, use 2 poached eggs, hollandaise sauce and slices of prosciutto.

Recipe #3: Cinnamon Sugar Donut Muffins

This recipe makes 12 muffins.

Ingredients –

- 2 large Eggs
- 2 tablespoons Psyllium Husk Powder
- 1/2 cup powdered Erythritol
- 1.5 cups Almond Flour
- 1/3 cup Salted Butter
- 1/2 cup Heavy Cream
- 1/2 teaspoon Orange Extract
- 1.5 teaspoons Baking Powder
- 1/4 teaspoon Allspice
- 1/8 teaspoon Ground Ginger
- 1/4 teaspoon Nutmeg
- 1/8 teaspoon Ground Clove
- 1/4 teaspoon Liquid Stevia
- For Cinnamon Sugar Coating
  - 1/4 cup melted Butter
  - 1 teaspoon Cinnamon
  - 1/4 cup Erythritol

Instructions –

- Take a small pan and place it on medium heat. Add 1/3rd cup butter to the pan. Let the butter melt.
- Using the grinder, grind clove twig and ½ cup Erythritol.
- Take a bowl and add all the dry Ingredients.
- By this time, the butter would have melted and turned golden brown. Set the pan aside for cooling.
- Once the butter has cooled down, add the dry Ingredients mix to it.
- Take a bowl and add all the wet Ingredients to the bowl. Beat well!
- To the beaten wet mix, add half of the dry Ingredients. Dough well and add the other half of the dry Ingredients to the wet mix.
- The oven must be set to preheat at 350 degrees Fahrenheit.
- Make small parts of the dough and put them into the cupcake molds.
- Put these molds in the oven and bake for around 25 minutes or until it is done.
- Let the molds cool down for around 10 minutes.
- Now that the muffins are done, it is time to prepare a sugar coating. For this, take a bowl and mix Erythritol and cinnamon.
- Take a pan and melt 1/4th cup butter on medium heat. Put the muffin into the butter and then into the cinnamon-sugar mix. You can either coat the whole muffin or just the muffin top.
- Allow the muffins to cool down and serve.

Recipe #4: Red Pepper, Bacon and Mozzarella Frittata

Serves – 6

Ingredients –

- 7 slices Bacon
- 1 medium Red Bell Pepper
- 4 large Bella Mushroom Caps
- 1/4 cup Heavy Cream
- 1/2 cup Chopped Fresh Basil
- 1/4 cup Parmesan Cheese, Grated
- ½ cup Goat Cheese, Grated
- 1 cup Fresh Mozzarella Cheese, Cubed
- 8-9 large Eggs
- 1 tablespoon Olive Oil
- Pepper (to taste)
- Salt (to taste)
- 2 tablespoon Fresh Parsley for garnishing

Instructions –

- Before starting, preheat the oven to 350 degrees Fahrenheit. Chop the red bell peppers, mushrooms and bacon.
- Take a pan and put 1-tablespoon olive oil in it. Once the olive oil heats up put the bacon in the pan. Fry the bacon until it becomes brown.
- Once the bacon turns brown, add the red bell peppers. Let the vegetables cook.
- Take a mixing bowl and add eggs, heavy cream, and pepper and Parmesan cheese to it. Mix the egg mixture well.
- Once the bell peppers are done, add the mushrooms and let it cook until it softens. Add basil at top.
- Now that the vegetables and bacon are done, add mozzarella cheese cubes.
- Pour the egg mixture on top and mix slightly to ensure that the egg mixture gets evenly distributed.
- Using a grater, grate the goat cheese and spread it on top of the frittata.
- Preheat the oven at 350 degrees Fahrenheit. Bake the frittata for 8 minutes.
- Next, put the frittata in the broiler and cook until the top becomes golden brown in color.
- Take the frittata on the pan out and allow it to rest for a minute.
- Remove the frittata from the pan onto a parchment paper, flip it and serve after garnishing it with parsley.

Recipe #5: Cinnamon Orange Scones

This recipe makes 8 scones.

Ingredients –

- Scones
    - Zest of 1 Orange
    - 2 Large Eggs
    - 2 tablespoon Maple Syrup
    - 1/4 Cup Cubes of Unsalted Butter
    - 1/4 Cup Erythritol
    - 1/3 Cup Heavy Cream
    - 1/2 Cup Coconut Flour
    - 1 tablespoon Golden Flaxseed
    - 1/4 teaspoon Stevia
    - 2 tablespoon Coconut Oil
    - 1.5 teaspoon Ground Cinnamon
    - 1/4 teaspoon Salt
    - 1.5 teaspoon Baking Powder
    - 1/4 teaspoon Xanthan Gum
    - 1 teaspoon Vanilla Extract
- Icing
    - 20 drops of Liquid Stevia
    - 1 tablespoon Orange Juice
    - 1/4 Cup Coconut Butter

Instructions –

- Put the oven to preheat at 400 degrees Fahrenheit.
- Take a bowl and put 7 tablespoons of coconut flour, baking powder, salt, coconut oil, golden flaxseed and orange zest. Mix well!
- Add cubed butter to this mix. Mixing this will create crumbled dough.
- Take another mixing bowl and using a hand mixer, mix liquid stevia, Erythritol and eggs.
- Once the eggs are well beaten, add vanilla extract, maple syrup and heavy cream. Beat the mix until the cream becomes thick.
- Add, to this mix, Xanthan Gum and Coconut flour.
- Keep a few tablespoons of the cream mixture aside. Put the rest of the cream mixture to the dough.
- Add cinnamon to the dough and knead the dough well.
- Flatten the dough and cut out 8 pizza-like slices of the dough.
- Put these slices on the parchment paper. Spread the remaining cream mixture on the slices using a brush. Sprinkle some cinnamon on top.
- Bake these slices for around 15 minutes.
- Let the scones cool down and ice them before serving.

Recipe #6: Shakshuka (Eggs poached in a spiced tomato sauce)

Serves – 4

Ingredients –

- 8 eggs
- 1 1/2 tbsp. ghee
- 4 medium tomatoes
- 1 large onion
- 1 small green bell pepper
- 1 small red bell pepper
- 2 Serrano pepper
- 4 cloves garlic
- 1 1/2 teaspoon paprika
- 1 1/2 tsp. cumin powder
- 1/4 tsp. chili powder
- Pepper to taste
- Salt to taste
- 2 tablespoons cilantro

Instructions –

- To start with, prepare all the vegetables and chop the onions. Also, chop the bell peppers, Serrano peppers, mince the garlic and dice the tomatoes.
- Take a large skillet and place it over medium heat. Add ghee to it. Allow it to melt. Add onions and sauté until light brown.
- Add garlic and Serrano pepper and sauté for a couple of minutes until fragrant. Add bell peppers and lower heat. Cook until bell peppers are soft.
- Add chili powder, paprika, cumin and sauté for a few seconds. Do not let the spices burn.
- Add tomatoes and simmer until sauce thickens. Add about 1/4 tsp. salt and mix.
- Make 8 small cavities in the sauce at different places in the skillet. Break an egg into each of the cavities.
- Sprinkle salt and pepper over it. Cover and simmer until the eggs are cooked. Cook the eggs as per your desire.
- Garnish with chopped cilantro and serve.

Recipe # 7: Swiss Chard & Ricotta Muffins / Pie

Serves – 6

Ingredients -

- 6 eggs, beaten
- 2 pounds mild sausages
- 1 large onion
- 2 cloves garlic
- 16 cups Swiss chard
- 2 tablespoons olive oil
- 4 cups whole milk ricotta cheese
- 1/2 cup parmesan cheese, shredded
- 2 cups mozzarella, shredded
- 1/4 teaspoon ground nutmeg
- Salt to taste
- Pepper powder to taste

Instructions –

- To start with, prepare the vegetables and chop the onions and Swiss chard. Also, mince the garlic.
- Take a large skillet and place it over medium heat. Add olive oil. When oil is heated, add onions and garlic and sauté until onions are translucent.
- Add Swiss chard and sauté until the leaves wilts.
- Add nutmeg, salt and pepper. Mix well and remove from heat. Let it cool for a while.
- Meanwhile, add all the 3 types of cheese to beaten eggs. Add Swiss chard and mix.
- For pie:
    - Take 2 pie tins and grease it with a little olive oil. Spread the sausages at the bottom of the tin and press it well.
    - Divide and pour the mixture into both the tins.
    - Bake in a preheated oven at 350 degree F for about 30 minutes or until well set. (You can bake in batches).
- For muffins:
    - Line the cups with the sausages. Pour the mixture into the lined muffin cups. Fill only up to 3/4 the cup.
    - Bake in a preheated oven at 350 degree F for about 30 minutes or until well set. (You can bake in batches).

Recipe # 8: Californian Chicken Omelet

Serves – 2

Ingredients –

- 4 slices bacon
- 1 small avocado, peeled, pitted
- 4 eggs
- 2 medium tomatoes
- 2 ounces deli cut chicken
- 2 teaspoon mustard
- 2 tablespoon mayonnaise
- Salt and pepper to taste

Instructions –

- Slice avocado and beat eggs.
- Take a nonstick pan and place it over medium heat. Add bacon and cook until brown. Remove from the pan. When cool enough to handle, slice the bacon and set aside.
- Place the same pan back on heat. Pour half the beaten egg into the pan. Sprinkle salt and pepper.
- When the eggs are half done, place half the chicken, half the bacon, half the avocado, and half the tomatoes on one half of the omelet.
- Fold the other half of the omelet over the filling part. Cover and cook until the eggs are cooked.
- Repeat the above 3 steps with the remaining Ingredients.
- Serve hot.

Recipe # 9: Smoked Salmon Frittata

Serves – 4

Ingredients –

- For smoked salmon frittata:
    - 8 large eggs
    - 1 teaspoon coconut oil or ghee
    - 7-8 ounces smoked salmon

- To serve:
    - 1 green onion
    - Green onion sauce as required

Instructions –

- Preheat the broiler before you start the preparations.
- Slice the green onion and beat eggs and set it aside.
- Take an ovenproof skillet and place it over medium heat. Add ghee. When ghee melts, add eggs and cook until the middle part is runny and sides are slightly set.
- Lay the smoked salmon on it. Place the skillet under the broiler and cook until the eggs are set.
- Remove from the oven. Garnish with green onions and serve with green onion sauce.

Recipe # 10: Turkey Breakfast Sausages

Serves – 3

Ingredients –

- 1 pound extra lean ground turkey breast
- 1/4 teaspoon cayenne pepper or to taste
- 1/2 teaspoon ground ginger
- 1/2 teaspoon sage
- 1/2 teaspoon salt or to taste
- 1/8 teaspoon pepper powder
- Cooking spray

Instructions –

- Add cayenne pepper, ginger, sage, salt, and pepper to a large bowl and mix well.
- Add ground turkey to the bowl and mix well using your hands. Mix until the mixture is well combined.
- Divide the mixture into 6 portions and shape into patties.
- Place a nonstick pan over medium heat. Spray with cooking spray.
- Place the patties on the pan and cook until the underside is brown. Flip sides and cook the other side too. The center of the patties should not be pink.
- Serve hot with a keto dip of your choice.

Recipe # 11: Breakfast Pizza Quiche

Serves – 6

Ingredients –

- 12 large eggs
- 2 cups mushrooms
- 2 green onions
- 3/4 cup roasted red peppers
- 2 teaspoons ghee
- 1/2 teaspoon dried oregano
- 3/4 teaspoon onion powder
- 3/4 teaspoon garlic powder
- 1/2 teaspoon black pepper
- 1/2 teaspoon sea salt
- 3 tablespoons pizza slices
- 4 1/2 ounces sliced pepperoni
- 1/3 cup coconut milk

Instructions –

- To start with, chop onions and slice mushrooms, green onions, and roasted red peppers. Quarter the pepperoni.
- Switch on the oven and preheat it to 375 degree F.
- Also grease a baking dish with a little melted ghee.
- Add eggs and coconut milk to a bowl and whisk well. Add garlic powder, onion powder, salt, pepper and oregano and whisk again until well combined.
- Add vegetables and pepperoni to it and stir.
- Pour this mixture into the prepared baking dish. Spread pizza sauce all over it.
- Place in the oven and bake for 25 minutes or until done.
- Remove from oven and cool for a while.
- Cut into wedges and serve.

Recipe # 12: Cream Cheese Pumpkin Pancake

Serves – 4

Ingredients –

- For the pumpkin butter:
    - 1 tablespoon pure pumpkin puree
    - 6 tablespoons butter, unsalted
    - 1/8 teaspoon stevia

- For the pancakes:
    - 4 ounces cream cheese
    - 4 eggs
    - 4 tablespoons coconut flour
    - 1/2 tablespoon pumpkin pie spice blend
    - 4 tablespoons butter

Instructions –

- To make the pumpkin butter:
    - Place butter and pumpkin in a microwavable dish. Mix well. Microwave for 10 seconds on high. Mix well. If not smooth, microwave for another 10 seconds.
    - When the pumpkin butter is smooth, add stevia and stir.
- To make the pancakes:
    - Add cream cheese, eggs, coconut flour and pumpkin pie spice to the blender. Blend until smooth. Transfer into a bowl.
    - Place a nonstick pan over medium heat. Add 1-tablespoon butter.
    - When the butter melts, pour about 1/4 of the batter. Swirl the pan a bit so that the pancake spreads.
    - Cook until the bottom side is golden brown. Flip sides and cook the other side until golden brown too.
    - Repeat the above 2 steps with the remaining batter.
    - To serve: Place a pancake on individual serving plates. Place a little of the pumpkin butter on the pancake and serve.

Recipe # 13: Bacon and Eggs

Serves – 2

Ingredients –

- 1 tbsp. salted butter
- 8 thick slices bacon
- 1 carrot, cleaned and peeled into strips
- ½ cup cauliflower or broccoli florets, chopped
- ½ cup celery, chopped finely
- ½ large onion, chopped
- 4 large eggs
- ½ cup Colby Jack or mature cheddar cheese, grated

Instructions –

- Cut the bacon into thin strips, cutting across the grain
- Melt the butter over a medium heat and add the bacon and the vegetables
- Sauté for about 20 minutes stirring often, until the bacon has started to go crispy on the edges and the vegetables are starting to caramelize
- Spread the bacon and vegetables evenly over the pan, well combined, and then, in each of the four quarters, make a dip in the mixture
- Break an egg into each of the dips and carry on cooking until the eggs are almost set. If you like your yolks cooked, place a lid over the pan and leave it to steam until the yolks are cooked through. If you like your yolks runny, cook until the white is set enough to flip the egg over and flash cook the other side
- Sprinkle cheese over the top of the bacon and eggs and allow to cook until the cheese has melted
- Serve hot

Recipe # 14: Lemon and Blueberry Muffins

Makes - 15 muffins

Ingredients –

- 2 cups of almond flour
- 1 cup of heavy cream
- 2 whole eggs
- 1/8 cup of butter, melted
- 5 packets of stevia or Splenda artificial sweetener
- ½ tsp. baking soda
- ½ tsp. dried lemon zest
- ½ tsp. lemon flavoring or extract
- ¼ tsp. salt
- 4 oz. blueberries, fresh not frozen

Instructions –

- Preheat your oven to 350° F
- Line the cups of a 15-count muffin pan with cupcake peppers. If you don't have a 15 count pan, use 12 count pans instead
- Mix the cream and the flour together
- Add in the eggs, one at a time and stir them in until mixed
- Add the sweetener, butter, flavorings, baking soda, and the spices to the bowl and mix them thoroughly
- Add the blueberries and carefully stir them in, distributing them throughout the batter evenly
- Divide the mixture between the 15 cases, filling each about half full
- Bake for 20 minutes or until the muffins have turned golden
- Leave to cool and serve with fresh butter

Recipe # 15: Egg Muffin Cups

Makes – 6 muffin cups

Ingredients –

- 6 whole eggs
- 6 slices of thin turkey ham, nitrate-free variety
- ½ cup sliced spinach
- 3 tbsp. chopped red bell pepper
- Mozzarella cheese, grated
- 2 tbsp. finely chopped red onion
- Fresh basil
- Salt and pepper

Instructions –

- Preheat your oven to 350° F
- Coat a non-stick muffin pan with olive oil spray
- Lay a slice of the turkey ham into each of the cups, allowing it to rest on the bottom and drape over the sides to make the cup a bit bigger
- Crack an egg into each cup
- Divide the chopped pepper, onion and spinach between the cup and sprinkle cheese over the top
- Season with the fresh basil, salt, and pepper
- Cook until the eggs have set and the whites have turned opaque – if you want runny yolks, about 10 minutes, 15 minutes for harder ones. Do keep in mind that these will continue to cook for a few minutes after you remove them from the oven

Recipe # 16: Choco Chia Pudding

Serves – 2

Ingredients –

- 3 tbsp. chia seeds
- 1 cup almond milk, unsweetened variety – you also use soy or full skim milk
- 1 scoop chocolate protein powder – you can use cocoa powder instead
- ¼ cup fresh or frozen raspberries
- Optional ingredient – 1 tsp. honey -not needed if you use protein powder

Instructions –

- Mix the milk and protein or cocoa powder together
- Add the chia seeds to the mix and stir well
- Leave the mixture to rest for 5 minutes and then stir well
- Leave for another 5 minutes and then stir again
- Leave in the refrigerator for 30 minutes and then serve with the raspberries on the top

Recipe # 17: Strawberry Chocolate Protein Shake

Serves - 1-2

Ingredients –

- 16 oz. almond milk, unsweetened
- 4 oz. heavy cream
- 2 scoops of chocolate whey protein powder
- 1 tbsp. strawberry syrup, sugar-free
- ½ cup crushed ice

Instructions –

- Add all the ingredients to your blender in the order of the recipe
- Blend until you have a smooth consistency
- Drink straight away or chill first

Recipe # 18: Cheese and Onion Quiche

Makes – 2 quiches

Ingredients –

- 6 cups of muenster and Colby jack cheese, shredded
- 2 tbsp. butter + extra for greasing the pans
- 1 large finely chopped onion
- 12 eggs
- 2 cups of heavy cream
- 1 tsp. salt
- 1 tsp. black pepper
- 2 tsp. dried thyme

Instructions –

- Preheat your oven to 350° F
- Melt the butter over a medium heat and sauté the vegetables until the onions are soft and translucent. Remove from the heat and leave to cool
- Grease 2 10" pie or quiche pans
- Add two cups of the shredded cheese to each one and the top off with the cooled vegetable mixture in an even layer
- Beat the eggs and add the cream and the spices. Whisk until thoroughly combined and the mixture is frothy
- Divide the mixture between the two pans and use a fork to gently distribute the vegetables and cheese evenly through the mixture
- Bake for 20 to 25 minutes, or until the mixture has set and is puffy, with a slight golden color to the center – test with a knife to see if the egg is set
- Serve hot

Can be refrigerated for up to one week or frozen for a later date.

Chapter 7: Lunch/Dinner Recipes

Diet plans can't show substantial results unless you add their elements in every facet of your eating. Lunch and dinner are the heaviest meals of the day and in order to help you add the right balance of nutrients to your ketogenic diet plan, we have given a list of delicious recipes for you to choose from.

Recipe #1: Skillet Chicken Pot Pie

Serves – 8

Ingredients –

- Crust
    - 1 large Egg
    - 1/4 cup Cream Cheese
    - 3 tablespoon Psyllium Husk Powder
    - 1/3 cup Almond Flour
    - 1/4 teaspoon Garlic Powder
    - 3 tablespoon Butter
    - 1/4 cup Cheddar Cheese
    - 1/2 teaspoon Paprika
    - 1/4 teaspoon Onion Powder
    - Salt and Pepper to Taste

- Filling
    - 5 slices Bacon
    - 6 small Chicken Thighs
    - 1 teaspoon Garlic Powder
    - 3/4 teaspoon Celery Seed
    - 1 teaspoon Onion Powder
    - 6 cups Spinach
    - 1 cup Cheddar Cheese
    - 1/4 cup Chicken Broth
    - 1 cup Cream Cheese
    - Pepper (to taste)
    - Salt (to taste)

Instructions –

- Remove the skin and bones from the chicken thighs. Cut the chicken into cubes and apply salt and pepper to it.
- Preheat the oven at 375 degrees Fahrenheit.
- Take a pan and season the chicken thighs with spices. Put the thighs in the oven and cook them until they turn brown.
- Take another pan and place sliced bacon in it. Cook the bacon until it turns brown.
- Take a pan and use chicken broth to de-glaze it. You must add cedar cheese and cream cheese to this pan. Keep stirring until the cheese melts.
- Put the spinach in the pan and allow it to wilt.

- Take a bowl and put all the dry Ingredients for making crust.
- In another bowl, add cream cheese and cedar cheese. Melt the cheese in the oven.
- To the dry Ingredients, add the egg and cheese mix. Form the Ingredients mix into a circle to form a crust. The crust should be the same size as the pan.
- Put all the Ingredients in the pan and invert the crust onto the pan.
- Allow the pan to cook in the oven at 375 degrees Fahrenheit for 15 minutes.
- The dish can be taken out and served.

Recipe #2: Buffalo Chicken Jalapeno Popper Casserole

Serves – 6

Ingredients –

- 6 slices Bacon
- 6 small Chicken Thighs
- 3 medium Jalapenos
- 1/4 cup Frank's Red Hot
- 1/4 cup Mayonnaise
- 1.5 cup Cream Cheese
- ½ cup Shredded Mozzarella Cheese
- 1 cup Shredded Cheddar
- Pepper (to taste)
- Salt (to taste)

Instructions –

- The first thing, before starting, is to debone the thighs. Next, preheat the oven at 400 degrees Fahrenheit.
- The second step is to season the chicken thighs with salt and paper.
- Now that the chicken thighs are ready, you can wrap them in a foil and place them on the rack for baking. They should be baked for 40 minutes.
- Take a pan and put it on medium heat.
- Take the bacon and make out 6 slices from it. Put the bacon on the pan for cooking.
- Once the bacon is cooked, it is time to add jalapenos to the pan.
- Wait until the jalapenos become soft and add Frank's Red Hot, mayo and cream cheese to the preparation.
- Mix all the Ingredients and add seasoning as per your requirements.
- Take the chicken thighs out and allow it to cool slightly.
- Place the chicken thighs in the casserole and spread the bacon mix to it.
- Garnish the dish with grated mozzarella and cheddar cheese.
- Bake the dish for 15 minutes and broil it for 5 minutes.
- Take it out and allow it to slightly cool down. Serve!

Recipe #3: Jalapeno Popper Soup

Serves – 6

Ingredients –

- 1 tablespoon Chicken Fat
- 3 medium Jalapenos, diced
- 4 medium Chicken Thighs
- 4 slices Bacon
- ¾ cup Cream Cheese
- 1 teaspoon Onion Powder
- 2 teaspoons Minced Garlic
- 1 teaspoon Dried Cilantro
- 1 cup Cheddar Cheese
- 3 cups Chicken Broth
- 1 teaspoon Cajun Seasoning
- Pepper (to taste)
- Salt (to taste)

Instructions –

- Preheat the oven to 400 degrees Fahrenheit. Be sure not to throw away the chicken bones.
- Add seasoning like salt and pepper to the deboned thighs.
- Put the thighs on the cooling rack of the oven and bake them for around 55 minutes.
- Take a pan and add chicken fat to it. Allow it to melt and then add chicken bones to it. Fry the bones for around 10 minutes.
- Add garlic, peppers and jalapenos to it. Cook until these vegetables become soft.
- Add the other spices and chicken broth and bring the broth to a boil. Once the broth begins to boil, slow down the heat to simmer and let the ensemble cook.
- By this time, the thighs would be done. Take the thighs out and allow it to slightly cool. Also, remove the bones from the broth.
- Add some extra chicken fat to the vegetables and puree the broth. Shred the chicken and add to the pot. Let it cook on simmer for 15 minutes.
- Add cheese and cream cheese to the soup and allow the cheese to melt.
- Take the slices of bacon and fry them until they become crisp.
- Serve the soup along with crisp bacon slices.

Recipe #4: Chicken Nuggets Served With Avocado Lime Dip

Serves – 4

Ingredients –

- The Nuggets
    - 1 large Egg
    - 1.5 oz. Pork Rinds
    - 8 Chicken Thighs
    - Zest of 1 Lime
    - 1/4 cup Flaxseed Meal
    - 1/4 teaspoon Salt
    - 1/8 teaspoon Cayenne Pepper
    - 1/4 cup Almond Meal
    - 1/8 teaspoon Garlic Powder
    - 1/4 teaspoon Chili Powder
    - 1/4 teaspoon Pepper
    - 1/8 teaspoon Onion Powder
    - 1/4 teaspoon Paprika

- The Sauce
    - 1/8 teaspoon Cumin
    - 1/2 cup Mayonnaise
    - 1/4 teaspoon Garlic Powder
    - 1/2 medium Hass Avocado
    - 1 tablespoon Lime Juice
    - 1/2 teaspoon Red Chili Flakes

Instructions –

- Take the chicken thighs and cut them small pieces. Set the oven on preheating at 400 degrees Fahrenheit.
- Take the food processor and add spices, zest of lime, pork rinds and almond and flaxseed meal. Mix until the mixture resembles fine crumbs. Put the mix in a bowl.
- Take a bowl and add the egg to it. Whisk the egg until no white can be separately seen. You may also add a little water.
- Take each of the chicken thigh pieces one-by-one. Put the piece first in the egg and then rub it over the crumbs so as to create a coating of the crumbs mix.
- Put the thigh pieces on the cookie sheet and spray some oil over it.
- All these nuggets to bake for 15 minutes or until the thigh pieces cook completely.
- In order to make the sauce, put all the Ingredients meant for a same in a bowl and mix well.
- Serve the nuggets with the sauce.

Recipe #5: Pepperoni Pizza

This recipe makes 6 slices of pizza.

Ingredients –

- Pizza Base
    - 1 large Egg
    - 3/4 cup Almond Flour
    - 1 tablespoon Italian Seasoning
    - 2 cups Mozzarella Cheese
    - 3 tablespoons Cream Cheese
    - 1 tablespoon Psyllium Husk Powder
    - 1/2 teaspoon Pepper
    - 1/2 teaspoon Salt

- Toppings
    - 1/2 cup Tomato Sauce
    - 1 cup Mozzarella Cheese
    - Oregano (for seasoning)
    - 16 slices Pepperoni

Instructions –

- Preheat the oven to 400 degrees Fahrenheit.
- Take a microwave safe bowl and put the mozzarella cheese in it. Put it in the oven and allow it to melt. Make sure that the cheese doesn't brown.
- Once the cheese is completely melted, which should not take more than 1.5 minutes, add egg and cream cheese to it. Mix well!
- To the cheese mixture, add salt, pepper, seasoning, almond flour and Psyllium husk powder. Keep mixing to avoid the formation of any lumps.
- Knead the dough well.
- Flatten the dough to form a circular base.
- Put the flattened pizza base in the oven and bake it for around 10 minutes. Then, flip the side and bake it for another 3-4 minutes.
- It is now time to put the toppings. So, put the pepperoni, tomato sauce and mozzarella cheese on the pizza base and bake it for 3-4 minutes or until the cheese melts nicely.
- When done, cut the pizza into slices, sprinkle with oregano and serve.

Recipe #6: Stuffed Poblano Peppers

This recipe makes 4 stuffed peppers.

Ingredients –

- 4 Poblano Peppers
- 1 teaspoon Chili Powder
- 1 lb. Ground Pork
- 1/4 cup Cilantro, packed
- 1/2 Small Onion
- 1 tablespoon Bacon Fat
- 1 Vine Tomato
- 1 teaspoon Cumin
- 7 Baby Bella Mushrooms
- Pepper (to taste)
- Salt (to taste)

Instructions –

- To start with, prepare all the vegetables and slice the mushrooms. Also, slice the onions, mince the garlic and dice the tomato.
- Take the poblano peppers, place them on a cookie sheet and broil them in the oven for 10 minutes. Be sure to flip and turn them, every 2-3 minutes, to ensure uniform cooking.
- Take the peppers out and remove their skin.
- Take a pan and put bacon fat in it. Allow it to melt. Sauté ground pork in this fat on medium high heat. Season the pork with salt and pepper.
- As the browning of the pork begins, push the pork to one side of the pan. Put cumin and chili powder in the pan. Also add the onions and garlic.
- Once the garlic and onion soften, add the mushrooms into the pan and mix well.
- When the mushrooms seem to absorb the fat in the pan, toss the tomatoes into the pan. Also, add the cilantro.
- Take the poblano peppers now and create a long slice in them, starting from the stem right to the bottom. Empty the seeds out and stuff the pork mixture into the peppers.
- Bake the stuffed peppers at 350 degrees Fahrenheit for close to 8 minutes.
- Serve them hot! You can also add a little more cheese to the dish, if you like.

Recipe #7: Crispy Curry Rubbed Chicken Thighs

This recipe makes 8 curry rubbed chicken thighs.

Ingredients –

- 1/4 Cup Olive Oil
- 8 Chicken Thighs (With Bones and Skin)
- 1.5 teaspoon Salt
- 1/4 teaspoon Ginger
- 2 teaspoon Yellow Curry
- 1/2 teaspoon All spice
- 1 teaspoon Ground Cumin
- 1/4 teaspoon Ground Cardamom
- 1/2 teaspoon Cayenne Pepper
- 1 teaspoon Paprika
- 1/2 teaspoon Chili Powder
- 1/4 teaspoon Ground Cinnamon
- 1 teaspoon Garlic Powder
- 1/2 teaspoon Ground Coriander

Instructions –

- Preheat the oven to 425 degrees Fahrenheit.
- This recipe requires a lot of spices. Get hold of all the spices, collect them and place them in such a manner that you can get them easily as and when you need them. You can take a big plate and take out the amount of spices you need in it so that you don't have to get hold of the bottles every now and then.
- In a bowl, mix all the spices mentioned in the Ingredients.
- Take the chicken thigh pieces and keep them on foil. Now, add around ½ spoon olive oil to each piece and apply the same on both sides of the thigh piece. Once the thigh piece has completely absorbed the olive on both sides, sprinkle spices mix over them. Carefully coat both sides of the piece with the spices mix.
- Put the thigh pieces on the cooling rack and bake them for 50 minutes.
- When you take out these baked chicken thigh pieces, you will see that the oil and spices, apart from what the piece has absorbed, is lying underneath the piece. When you place the chicken for serving, you can spoon this mix out and pour it over the piece for extra flavor.
- For garnishing, you may pour chives and red pepper flakes and serve.

Recipe #8: Cobb Salad

Serves – 2

Ingredients –

- For the dressing:
    - 2 tablespoons olive oil
    - 2 tablespoons apple cider vinegar
    - 2 teaspoons lemon juice
    - 2 teaspoons Dijon mustard
    - 1 clove garlic, minced
    - Salt to taste
    - Pepper powder to taste

- For the salad:
    - Cooking spray
    - 1 cup ham
    - 8 cherry tomatoes
    - 1/4 cup blue cheese, shredded
    - 4 hard-boiled eggs
    - 4 cups romaine lettuce
    - 1 avocado, peeled, pitted
    - 4 slices turkey bacon

Instructions –

- To make dressing: Add oil, vinegar, lemon juice, mustard, garlic, salt and pepper to a bottle with a lid. Fasten the lid and shake until well combined. Keep aside until use.
- To make salad:
    - Firstly chop ham into cubes. Slice the eggs. Chop lettuce and avocado.
    - Place a pan over medium heat. Spray with cooking spray. Add the ham and cook for about 5 minutes. Remove from heat and keep aside.
    - Place the lettuce at the bottom of a large salad bowl.
    - Lay the tomatoes, avocado, blue cheese, ham, eggs and bacon in rows.
    - Sprinkle the dressing all over the salad and serve.

Recipe #9: Peri Peri Chicken Salad

Serves – 4

Ingredients –

- 2 chicken breasts
- 4 pieces bacon
- 8 cups baby spinach
- 2 small avocadoes, pitted
- 4 tablespoons peri peri sauce

Instructions –

- Firstly slice the avocadoes. Chop bacon into bite sized pieces. Slice chicken breasts.
- Place skillet over medium heat. Add bacon and cook until crisp and nicely browned.
- Remove bacon with a slotted spoon. (There will be fat remaining in the pan)
- Add chicken slices to the same pan and cook on both the sides until done.
- Place spinach in a large salad bowl. Place avocado slices over it,
- Next lay the bacon over it. Drizzle peri peri sauce and serve.

Recipe # 10: Salmon Salad

Serves – 4

Ingredients –

- 3 stalks celery
- 2 shallots
- 2 cloves of garlic
- 1 bell pepper
- 1 medium cucumber
- 1/2 pint tomatoes
- 1/4 olive oil or to taste
- Juice of 1/2 a lemon
- Zest of 1/2 a lemon
- 1 tablespoon red wine vinegar
- 1/2 teaspoon kosher salt or to taste
- 1/2 teaspoon fresh or dried dill
- 1/4 teaspoon freshly ground black pepper
- 1/4 teaspoon smoked paprika
- 1/4 teaspoon ground cumin
- 1/4 teaspoon crushed red pepper flakes
- 2 cans salmon, drained

Instructions –

- Thinly slice celery and bell pepper. Mince shallots and garlic. Halve the cucumber lengthwise and then slice it. Halve the tomatoes
- Add all the Ingredients to a large bowl. Toss well and refrigerate for an hour.
- Taste and adjust the seasoning if necessary and serve.

Recipe # 11: Cream of Mushroom Soup

Serves – 2

Ingredients –

- 3 cups cauliflower florets
- 2 cups unsweetened almond milk
- 1 1/2 teaspoons onion powder
- 1/2 teaspoon Himalayan rock salt
- Freshly ground pepper, to taste
- 1 teaspoon extra-virgin olive oil
- 2 1/2 cups white mushrooms
- 1 yellow onion
- 1/2 teaspoon garlic powder

Instructions –

- Chop onions and set aside.
- Add garlic, cauliflower, milk, onion powder, salt and pepper to a saucepan.
- Place the pan over medium heat. Bring to a boil.
- Lower heat and simmer until the cauliflowers are soft. Remove from heat and puree the cauliflower using an immersion blender.
- Meanwhile, place a saucepan over medium heat. Add oil. When the oil is heated, add onions and sauté for a couple of minutes. Add mushrooms and sauté until the onions are light brown.
- Add the cauliflower puree. Mix well and bring to a boil.
- Reduce heat and simmer for 10-12 minutes. If you find the soup too thick, add some more milk and heat thoroughly.
- Ladle into individual soup bowls and serve hot.

Recipe # 12: Chicken Soup

Serves – 4

Ingredients –

- 1/2 pound chicken, cleaned, rinsed
- 1 medium zucchini
- 1 medium carrot, peeled
- 1 medium onion
- 1 teaspoon garlic powder
- 4 cups water or chicken stock
- 1/2 tablespoons chicken soup powder
- 1 teaspoon turmeric powder
- 1 tablespoon fresh dill
- Salt to taste
- Pepper powder to taste

Instructions –

- Firstly prepare the vegetables. Grate carrot and zucchini. Chop onion into chunks. Chop dill.
- Take a saucepan and place it over medium heat. Add stock or water and let it boil.
- Add chicken, onion, garlic powder, soup powder, dill, turmeric, salt and pepper.
- Let it cook until tender. Remove the chicken pieces from the saucepan with a slotted spoon and set aside on a plate. When cool enough to handle, shred the meat and add it back to the saucepan.
- Add vegetables and simmer for 8-10 minutes.
- Ladle into bowls and serve.

Recipe # 13: Beef and Vegetable Soup

Serves – 8

Ingredients –

- 12 cups beef stock
- 2 medium turnips, peeled,
- 1 daikon radish,
- 1 baby bok Choy
- 1 medium onion
- 2 cups portabella mushrooms
- 1 cup zucchini,
- 1/2 cup cremini mushrooms,
- 1 1/4 pounds, beef stew meat, chopped into small pieces
- 1/2 tablespoon oil
- Salt to taste
- Pepper powder to taste

Instructions –

- Firstly chop beef into small pieces. Finely chop turnips, radish, bok Choy, Portabella mushrooms, cremini mushrooms, and zucchini. Chop onions.
- Take a large saucepan and place it over medium heat. Add stock, turnip, radish, and bok Choy.
- Meanwhile place a frying pan over medium heat. Add oil and sauté the onions until brown. Transfer into the saucepan.
- Add cremini mushrooms to the same frying pan and sauté until brown. Transfer to the saucepan.
- Add mushrooms to the same frying pan and sauté until brown. Transfer to the saucepan.
- Add meat to the same frying pan and sauté until brown. Transfer to the saucepan.
- Bring to a boil. Lower heat, cover and simmer for a couple of hours until the meat is cooked. Season with salt and pepper.
- Ladle into soup bowls and serve

Recipe # 14: Keto Beef Stir Fry

Serves – 2

Ingredients –

- 1 tbsp. coconut oil
- ½ medium Spanish onion
- 5 brown mushrooms
- 2 large kale leaves
- ½ cup broccoli
- ½ medium red bell pepper
- 10 ½ oz. ground beef
- 1 tbsp. Chinese Five Spices
- 1 tbsp. cayenne pepper

Instructions –

- Chop up the broccoli, kale, onion and pepper and slice up the mushrooms
- Heat the coconut oil over a medium-high heat in a large skillet and sauté the onions for about a minute
- Add in the rest of the chopped vegetables and cook, stirring constantly, for about 2 minutes
- Add in the ground beef, the spices, stir to combine and cook for about 2 minutes
- Turn the heat down to medium, cover the pan and leave to cook for about 5 or 10 minutes, until the beef is brown
- Serve hot, on its own or with cauliflower rice

Recipe # 15: Ginger Beef

Serves – 2

Ingredients –

- 2 4 oz. sirloin steaks, sliced into strips
- 1 tbsp. extra virgin olive oil
- 1 small diced onion
- 1 clove crushed garlic
- 2 small tomatoes, diced
- 1 tsp. ground ginger
- 4 tbsp. apple cider vinegar
- Salt and pepper for seasoning

Instructions –

- Heat the oil in a large skillet over a medium-high heat and brown off the steak trips
- When both sides of the meat are seared, add the tomatoes, garlic, and onions
- In a separate bowl, mix the ginger with the vinegar and season with salt and pepper – add to the skillet with the meat and vegetables
- Stir well to combine cover the pan and reduce the heat down to low. Simmer until the liquid has completely evaporated
- Serve hot

Recipe # 16: Baked Salmon

Serves – 2

Ingredients –

- 2 6 oz. salmon fillets
- 2 cloves minced garlic
- 6 tbsp. olive oil
- 1 tsp. salt
- 1 tsp. dried basil
- 1 tsp. black pepper
- 1 tbsp. fresh lemon juice
- 1 tbsp. fresh chopped parsley

Instructions –

- Make the marinade by combining the olive oil garlic, salt, basil, pepper, parsley and lemon juice together in a glass bowl
- Lay the salmon fillets into a glass baking dish and pour the marinade over the top
- Refrigerate for 60 minutes, turning the salmon occasionally to coat thoroughly
- Preheat your oven to 375° F
- Remove the salmon from the marinade and place onto foil
- Pour marinade over the top and wrap the salmon up folding the edges over to create a sealed pocket
- Bake for 35 to 45 minutes or until the salmon is flaky

Recipe # 17: Spinach, Tomato, and Sardine Soup

Serves - 2

Ingredient –

- 2 tbsp. cold pressed corn or vegetable oil
- 1 tbsp. crushed garlic
- 1 whole onion, sliced
- 1 large tomato, sliced
- 1 can (4 3/8 o) sardines in olive oil and tomato sauce
- 2-3 cups vegetable broth or water
- 1-2 cups fresh spinach leaves
- 1 tsp. salt
- 1 tsp. ground black pepper

Instructions –

- Heat the oil over a medium-high heat
- Sauté the onion, garlic, and tomato for about 3 to 5 minutes, or until the tomatoes and onions are soft
- Add the sardines and stir well to combine. Crush them into small pieces so they soak up the flavor of the tomatoes and onion
- Add the broth or water and bring to the boil. Reduce the heat to a simmer
- Add the spinach, season with the salt and pepper and stir well
- Cook for 1 or 2 minutes until the spinach has softened but not wilted
- Serve hot

Recipe # 18: Reuben Casserole

Serves – 2

Ingredients –

- ½ lb. corned beef
- 1 can sauerkraut, drained thoroughly
- 2 cups shredded Swiss cheese
- ½ cup full fat mayonnaise
- 8 oz. cream cheese
- ½ cup ketchup – low sugar variety
- 2 tbsp. pickle brine
- ½ tsp. caraway seed

Instructions –

- Preheat your oven to 350° F
- Melt the mayonnaise, cream cheese and ketchup together, stirring to combine over a low heat
- While it melts, dice your corned beef into chunks of about ½ inch
- Add the drained sauerkraut to the cream cheese mix; add in 1½ cups of the cheese and the corned beef. Cook, stirring until the cheese has melted and all the ingredients are combined
- Remove the sauce from the heat and add the pickle brine. If you don't have any of this you can add 1 tsp of vinegar, 1 tbsp. salt and a small pinch of garlic powder
- Pour the mixture into a greased pan and sprinkle the rest of the grated cheese over the top
- Garnish with the caraway seeds and bake for about 20 minutes, or until the cheese on the top has melted and the casserole is bubbling
- Serve hot

Recipe # 19: Butter Paneer Curry

Serves – 4

Ingredients –

- 3 lbs. bone-in chicken thigh
- 7 oz. paneer
- 1 cup of water
- 1 cup of crushed tomato
- ½ cup of heavy whipping cream
- 4 tbsp. of salted butter
- 1 tbsp. of olive oil
- 2 tsp of coconut oil
- 1 ½ tsp of garlic paste
- 1 ½ tsp of ginger paste
- 1 tsp of coriander powder
- 1 tsp of garam masala
- 1 tsp of salt
- 1 tsp of black pepper
- ½ tsp of paprika
- ½ tsp of red chili powder
- ½ tsp of Kashmiri Mirch
- 5 sprigs of fresh cilantro

Instructions –

- Preheat your oven to 375° F
- Rub the olive oil over the chicken and season with salt and pepper
- Roast the chicken for about 25 minutes
- Chop the paneer into small bits and set to one side
- Heat the coconut oil and butter over a medium heat until the butter begins to brown
- Add the garlic and ginger pastes, stir and sauté for about 2 minutes
- Add the tomato, garam masala, coriander powder, chili powder, paprika, and salt. Stir well and leave to simmer until you see oil beginning to form on the top
- Mix the paneer into the sauce gently
- Add the water and leave to simmer for about 5 minutes
- Add the cream and turn the heat to medium low, stirring to mix
- Leave t simmer until it starts to boil
- Take the chicken off the bone and add the meat to the sauce (the chicken should NOT be fully cooked at this point)
- Simmer for about 5 minutes
- Serve hot garnished with fresh cilantro.

Chapter 8: Dessert Recipes

This chapter includes ten dessert recipes that can be included into your ketogenic diet plan. You can choose any of these recipes depending on the availability of Ingredients and personal preferences. You will notice that these recipes make extensive use of natural sweeteners because of the health benefits associated with them. You can replace the sweetener with any natural sweetener of your choice and add in the amounts that you prefer.

Recipe #1: Gelatin Pudding

Serves – 2

Ingredients –

- 2 tablespoon water
- 2 tablespoon cocoa powder
- 1 tablespoon gelatin
- 2 tablespoon honey
- 1 cup coconut milk (canned, full fat)

Instructions -

- Put a pan on medium heat and add honey, cocoa and coconut milk. Keep whisking!
- Take a small bowl and add water and gelatin to it. Mix well!
- Add the gelatin mixture to the pan.
- Take two pudding cups and put the mixture of coconut milk into them.
- Freeze the cups for more than 30 minutes.

Recipe #2: Coconut Oil Candies

Ingredients –

- 2 tablespoons almond butter
- 1/2 teaspoon Celtic Sea Salt
- 2 tablespoons organic cocoa powder (unsweetened)
- 1 cup softened virgin coconut oil (cold pressed)
- 1 tablespoon sweetener
- 1 teaspoon vanilla extract
- Desiccated Coconut

Instructions -

- Take a bowl and add in all the Ingredients. Mix well! You may also make a smooth mixture by putting all the Ingredients into the blender.
- Make candies by taking spoonsful of the mixture and putting it in desiccated coconut or on butter paper.
- Put the candies in for refrigeration and take them out once they become solid.

Recipe #3: Berries and Whipped Coconut Cream

Serves – 2

Ingredients –

- Berries
- Optional: Dark chocolate
- 1 Can Coconut Milk (Full Fat, Unsweetened)

Instructions –

- Put the can of coconut milk in the refrigerator overnight.
- The next day, take out the thick layer of coconut milk, leaving out the water.
- Take a whisker and whip the coconut milk extracted from the can.
- Add in the berries.
- Although, this is optional, you can also add in some chocolate shavings, as garnishing, for people who like chocolate.

Recipe #4: Sugar-free Lemon Curd

Serves – 1

Ingredients –

- 2 large eggs
- 2 large egg yolks
- 2 tablespoon + 2 teaspoon Sweetener
- ½ Cup Lemon Juice
- 6 tablespoons butter cubes

Instructions –

- Take a saucepan and whisk in egg yolks, eggs, lemon juice and sweetener.
- Put the pan on the burner, add the butter and cook on low heat. Be sure to keep the heat very low or you will end up making a lemony egg scramble.
- You can switch the heat to medium-high after all the butter has melted.
- Stir regularly and cook until the mixture become thick enough to be compared to the conditioner.
- Strain the mixture through a fine strainer. This will remove bits of egg, leaving a smooth mixture. You can put this mixture in the fridge for later use.

Recipe #5: Brownie Cheese Cake

Serves – 10

Ingredients –

- Filling for Cheesecake:
    - ½ cup Sweetener
    - ½ teaspoon vanilla extract
    - ¼ cup heavy cream
    - 2 large eggs
    - 2 cups softened Cream Cheese
    -
- Base for Brownie:
    - ½ cup almond flour
    - 2 large eggs
    - ½ cup butter
    - ¼ cup cocoa powder
    - ¾ cup Sweetener
    - ½ cup chocolate (unsweetened and chopped)
    - ¼ teaspoon vanilla extract
    - ¼ cup chopped walnuts
    - A pinch of salt

Instructions –

- Preheat the oven to 325 degrees Fahrenheit.
- Take a spring-form pan and butter it. Also, cover its bottom with foil.
- Take a bowl and add in butter and chocolate. Melt these together by putting them in the microwave for half a minute. Be sure to take a microwave-safe bowl. Mix the melted chocolate until it becomes smooth.
- Take a small bowl and add salt, cocoa powder and almond flour in it.
- Take another bowl and add eggs and vanilla extract. Beat the mixture!
- Add the almond flour mix to the beaten eggs. Keep on mixing to avoid any crumbs. Finally, once the mixture is smooth, add the nuts.
- Place the mix into the buttered pan and bake it for 15-20 minutes.
- Let the baked brownie cool down for 15-20 minutes.
- Now that the base is ready, it is time to make the filling. Bring the temperature of the oven down to 300 degrees Fahrenheit.
- Take a bowl and whisk in cream cheese and eggs. Also, add in vanilla extract.
- Pour this filling into the crust. Take a large cookie sheet and put the cheesecake on it. Bake this cheesecake for 35-40 minutes and allow it to cool.
- Take the cake out by running the knife through the edges. Refrigerate this cake for a few hours after covering it with a plastic wrap.
- Serve this cake with chocolate sauce.

Recipe # 6: Chocolate Chip and Caramel Mini Muffins

Makes – 45 mini muffins

Ingredients –

- 2 cups of almond flour
- 1/8 cup of Erythritol sweetener
- ½ tsp baking soda
- ½ tsp xanthan gum
- ½ tsp salt
- 2 large eggs
- 1 cup sour cream
- 2 tbsp. melted, slightly cooked butter
- 1 tsp stevia glycerite
- ½ cup caramel dip
- ¾ cup chocolate chips – semi-sweet, made with cocoa powder

Instructions –

- Preheat your oven to 350° F
- Use paper liners to line to 45 mini muffin cups
- Whisk the flour, erythritol salt, gum and baking soda together
- Beat the eggs in a separate bowl, add the cream, stevia and butter and whisk together
- Add the wet mixture to the flour mix and stir in well
- Pour the batter into the muffin cups, filling them about ¾ full
- Bake for about 20 or 25 minutes or until the muffins have gone light brown and are springy
- Remove from the oven and leave to cool before removing them from the paper
- Serve with cream or refrigerate

Recipe # 7: Lemon Cheesecake

Serves – 4

Ingredients –

- 8 oz. softened cream cheese
- 2 oz. heavy cream
- 1 tsp stevia glycerite
- 1 tsp Splenda or another low carb sweetener
- 1 tbsp. fresh lemon juice
- 1 tsp vanilla flavoring

Instructions –

- Mix everything together in one bowl until you have a mixture the consistency of pudding
- Spoon the mixture into small cups or dishes and refrigerate to set
- Serve chilled with shredded coconut sprinkled over the top.

Chapter 9:
Low Carb Smoothies

Recipe # 1: Chocolate Peppermint Smoothie

Serves – 1

Ingredients –

- I cup cashew milk
- 1 scoop chocolate whey protein powder
- ¼ tsp mint extract
- A good handful of spinach
- Ice

Instructions –

- Place all the ingredients into your blender
- Blend until smooth

Recipe # 2: Peanut Butter Smoothie

Serves – 1

Ingredients –

- 1 scoop chocolate whey protein powder
- 1 cup water
- 1/3 cup heavy cream
- 2 tbsp. organic peanut butter
- 2 ice cubes

Instructions –

- Place all of the ingredients into a blender, liquid first
- Blend until smooth

Recipe # 3: Sage and Strawberry Smoothie

Serves – 1

Ingredients –

- 1 cup coconut milk, unsweetened
- 5 frozen strawberries
- 1 fresh sage leaf
- 2 tbsp. heavy cream
- 1 tbsp. vanilla syrup, sugar-free

Instructions –

- Blend all the ingredients together until smooth
- Drink straight away or chill first

Recipe # 4: Creamy Egg Smoothie

Serves – 1

Ingredients –

- 2 whole eggs, raw
- 2 tbsp. cream cheese
- ¼ cup heavy cream
- 1 tbsp. vanilla syrup, sugar-free
- 3 ice cubes

Instructions –

- Beat the eggs and add to the blender
- Add the rest of the ingredients and blend until smooth

Recipe # 5: Raspberry Cheesecake Smoothie

Serves – 1

Ingredients –

- 1 cup almond milk, unsweetened
- ½ cup fresh or frozen thawed raspberries
- 1 oz. cream cheese
- 1 tbsp. vanilla syrup, sugar-free

Instructions –

- Blend all the ingredients together until a smooth creamy consistency
- Chill for 30 minutes before drinking or add ice to chill it straightaway

Recipe # 6: Strawberries and Cream Smoothie

Serves – 1

Ingredients –

- 5 fresh or frozen strawberries
- 1 tbsp. vanilla syrup, sugar-free
- 3 tbsp. heavy cream

Instructions –

- Blend the ingredients together on high power
- Chill or add ice to drink straight away

Recipe # 7: Choco-Orange Smoothie

Serves – 1

Ingredients –

- 1 cup cashew milk
- 1 scoop chocolate whey protein powder
- 1/8 tsp orange extract
- A good handful of fresh spinach
- Ice

Instructions –

- Add the ingredients to the blender in the recipe order
- Blend until smooth and creamy

Recipe # 8: Strawberry Chocolate Smoothie

Serves – 1

Ingredients –

- 1 cup water
- 1 scoop chocolate whey protein powder
- 3 strawberries, frozen
- 3 tbsp. heavy cream

Instructions –

- Blend the ingredients together until smooth and creamy
- Add ice or chill first

Chapter 10:
Tips for Losing Weight

The reason why ketogenic diets are effective lies in the functional property of fat adaption. Your body needs to be told that it has to derive its energy from fats. The biggest challenge in this regard is to keep the body programmed to this state, on a regular basis. In order to maintain ketosis, here are a few tips that you must pay heed to.

Tip #1: Drink Enough Water

You must drink a healthy amount of water to maintain a healthy body. This is a fact that all of us know and are told about time and again. However, it has also proven to be the most difficult advice to follow. The modern lifestyle is so consuming that we mostly forget simple things like keeping our bodies hydrated and eating our meals on time. It is a good idea to drink around 4 glasses of water, first thing in the morning and another 4 glasses of water before the clock strikes noon.

Tip #2: Fast Once In A While

Like we said, our bodies fail to use up the fat stores because we never, ever fast. The body is pre-programmed to run ketosis as and when the body starves. Therefore, if you are finding it hard to get your body into ketosis or maintain the ketosis state of the body, you can fast intermittently. Fasting also helps in reducing food intake and manages appetites and cravings, both of which are crucial for your diet plan. However, be sure to go on a low-carb diet for a few days before fasting intermittently. The sudden lack of sugar in the body may land you up in a hypoglycemic state.

A daylong fast can be easily broken down into two phases. The first phase extends from the first meal you consume to the last meal you eat for the day. This is the build-up phase. The second phase, which extends from your last meal for the day to the first meal of the next day, is the cleansing phase. Ideally, the cleansing phase must be longer than the build-up phase. Whenever you fast, be sure to keep your body hydrated and eat good fats like butter and coconut oil. These additions play an instrumental role in boosting up the ketone production of the body and help to maintain a healthy insulin level.

Tip #3: Add Good Salts

The high insulin levels of the body, when it is in glycolysis, effect the functioning of the kidney in such a manner that the body retains sodium. As a result, the sodium-potassium ratio destabilizes. This is why most people are advised to reduce their sodium intake. On the other hand, when on a ketogenic diet, the insulin levels are normal and the kidney functioning allows sodium excretion more effectively.

As a result, the body needs sodium to ensure proper functioning. Never make the mistake of avoiding salts when running your body on a ketogenic diet. There are several ways by which you can increase the sodium levels of the body. Some of the best ways include having broth, eating sprouted pumpkin seeds, eating cucumber as part of the salad for natural sodium and adding a pinch of salt to almost everything you eat.

Tip #4: Exercise

Regular exercise can play a crucial role in maintaining the ketosis state of the body and avoiding deposition of glucose in body parts. Exercise allows activation of glucose transport molecules that facilitate deposition of glucose in the muscles and liver. Exercises like the ones used for resistance training also facilitate maintenance of normal blood sugar levels.

It is important to understand in this context that overdoing exercise can result in the release of stress hormones. This, in turn, increases sugar levels of the body and destabilizes the ketosis state of the body. Regular and 'just-enough' exercise can be a great way to keep you on track.

Tip #5: Avoid Too Much Protein

Most regular diet programs recommend higher protein intake. However, excessive protein intake can initiate what is called gluconeogenesis, which again generates glucose. If you feel that your body is no longer able to maintain the ketosis state, you must take a keen look at the amount of proteins that you are consuming. You may have more success with a much lower protein intake.

Tip #6: Choose What You Eat Wisely

Although ketogenic diet recommends a reduced carbohydrate intake, it is not a good idea to remove carbs from the diet completely. Therefore, inclusion of starchy vegetables and citric fruits is a good idea. On an odd day when you are off-ketosis, you can consume berries and potatoes. However, when on ketosis, be sure to avoid sweet potato and berry-type fruits completely.

Tip #7 Reduce Stress

Stress is the root cause of most of the problems that your body's face. In fact, an increase in the stress hormones in the body can pull you off ketosis because it increases the sugar levels substantially. Therefore, maintaining a ketosis state can be an uphill task if you are going through stressful times in your life. Managing stress is an important facet of the ketogenic diet. Adopt strategies that keep your stress levels in check if you wish to make your ketogenic diet work. In line with this objective, having adequate amounts of daily sleep and maintaining a stable lifestyle are also essential.

Conclusion

Ketogenic diet is a great diet program for people who find it hard to keep away from fatty foods and tempting recipes. This diet plan allows you to consume all the butter and oil in the world yet keep you within the limit as far as weight is concerned. However, there are several challenges and limitations that exist as far as getting into and remaining in the ketosis state.

This book contains carefully picked recipes for all the different courses of the meal to help you include the ketogenic diet as easily as possible. You can go ahead and try these recipes to make a menu-plan for yourself. Besides this, there are some proven tips for you to adopt and implement as part of your lifestyle.

The right lifestyle is absolutely essential for maintaining the ketosis state. In addition to getting the diet right, it is equally important to maintain and manage your stress level, get the right amount of sleep, and have the mental alertness and clarity to overcome appetite bursts and sugar cravings.

In order to get this correct, you need to understand your body and how it responds to changes in diet and lifestyle. This will help you understand the factors that are essential for keeping your body in ketosis or are responsible for knocking you out of ketosis. Understand your body; change your lifestyle; eat right for a healthier and happier life.